AIDS TO THE EXAMINATION OF THE PERIPHERAL NERVOUS SYSTEM

SIXTH EDITION

AIDS TO THE EXAMINATION OF THE PERIPHERAL NERVOUS SYSTEM

ISBN: 978-0-3238-7110-5

Publisher: Jeremy Bowes
Content Project Manager: Shubham Dixit
Design: Brian Salisbury
Illustration Coordinator: Narayanan Ramakrishnan
Marketing Manager: Deborah Watkins

 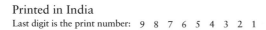

Working together
to grow libraries in
developing countries

www.elsevier.com • www.bookaid.org

Printed in India
Last digit is the print number: 9 8 7 6 5 4 3 2 1

In 1940 Dr George Riddoch was Consultant Neurologist to the Army. He realised the necessity of providing centres to deal with peripheral nerve injuries during the war. In collaboration with Professor J. R. Learmonth, Professor of Surgery at the University of Edinburgh, peripheral nerve injury centres were established in the neurosurgical units at Gogarburn near Edinburgh and at Killearn near Glasgow. Professor Learmonth suggested an illustrated guide on peripheral nerve injuries for the use of surgeons working in general hospitals. In collaboration with Dr Ritchie Russell, a few photographs demonstrating the testing of individual muscles were taken in 1941. Dr Russell returned to Oxford in 1942 and was replaced by Dr M. J. McArdle as Neurologist to Scottish Command. The photographs were completed by Dr McArdle at Gogarburn with the help of the Department of Medical Illustration at the University of Edinburgh. About 20 copies in loose-leaf form were circulated to surgeons in Scotland.

In 1942 Professor Learmonth and Dr Riddoch added the diagrams illustrating the innervation of muscles by various peripheral nerves modified from Pitres and Testut (*Les Neufs en Schemas*, Doin, Paris, 1925) and the diagrams of cutaneous sensory distributions and dermatomes. This was first published by the Medical Research Council in 1942 as *Aids to the Investigation of Peripheral Nerve Injuries* (War Memorandum No. 7) and revised in 1943. It became a standard work, and over the next 30 years many thousands of copies were printed.

It was thoroughly revised between 1972 and 1975 with new photographs and many new diagrams, including a coloured drawing of the brachial plexus, and was republished under the title *Aids to the Examination of the Peripheral Nervous System* (Memorandum No. 45), reflecting the wide use made of this booklet by students and practitioners and its more extensive use in clinical neurology, which was rather different from the wartime emphasis on nerve injuries.

In 1984 the Medical Research Council transferred responsibility for this publication to the Guarantors of *Brain* for whom a new edition was prepared. Modifications were made to some of the diagrams, and a new drawing of the lumbosacral plexus was included.

Most of the photographs for the 1943, 1976 and 1986 editions show Dr. McArdle, who died in 1989, as the examining physician. A new set of colour photographs was prepared for the fourth edition published in 2000 with Dr. M. D. O'Brien as the examining physician. The diagrams of the brachial plexus and lumbosacral plexus were retained, but all other diagrams were redrawn, including the cutaneous branches. The introduction for the fifth edition, published in 2010, was revised and new diagrams of the cutaneous distribution of the trigeminal nerve added. New to this edition are a diagram of the spine and spinal roots, a list of the common entrapment and compression palsies with arrows to show these sites in the peripheral nerve diagrams, and new diagrams of the dermatome and nerve distribution of the male inguinal region and the female perineum. The nerve diagrams are not intended to illustrate anatomic detail but to show the usual order of innervation so that the level of a lesion can be determined; the usual pattern is shown, but there is considerable variation in the branching patterns of peripheral nerves (Sunderland 1978). There have been a few minor changes to existing diagrams.

M.D. O'Brien
for The Guarantors of *Brain*

Sunderland S. *Nerve and Nerve Injuries*. 2nd ed. London: Churchill Livingstone; 1978.
See Compston A. From the archives. *Brain* 2010;133:2838–2844 for a detailed account of the history of this publication.

MRC Nerve Injuries Committee, 1942–1943

Brigadier G. Riddoch, MD, FRCP *(Chairman)*
Brigadier W. Rowley Bristow, MB, FRCS
G. L. Brown, MSc, MB *(1942)*
Brigadier H. W. B. Cairns, DM, FRCS
E. A. Carmichael, CBE, MB, FRCP
Surgeon Captain M. Critchley, MD, FRCP, RNVR
J. G. Greenfield, MD, FRCP
Professor J. R. Learmonth, CBE, ChM, FRCSE
Professor H. Platt, MD, FRCS
Professor H. J. Seddon, DM, FRCS *(1942)*
Air Commodore C. P. Symonds, MD, FRCP
J. Z. Young, MA
F. J. C. Herrald, MB, MRCPE *(Secretary)*

MRC Revision Subcommittee, 1972–1975

Sir Herbert Seddon, CMG, DM, FRCS *(Chairman until October 1973)*
Professor J. N. Walton, TD, MD, DSc, FRCP *(Chairman from October 1973)*
Professor R. W. Gilliatt, DM, FRCP
M. J. F. McArdle, MB, FRCP
M. D. O'Brien, MD, MRCP
Professor P. K. Thomas, DSc, MD, FRCP
R. G. Willison, DM, FRCPE

Editorial Committee for the Guarantors of Brain, 1984–1986

Sir John Walton, TD, MD, DSc, FRCP *(Chairman)*
Professor R. W. Gilliatt, DM, FRCP
M. Hutchinson, MB, BDS
M. J. F. McArdle, MB, FRCP
M. D. O'Brien, MD, FRCP
Professor P. K. Thomas, DSc, MD, FRCP
R. G. Willison, DM, FRCPE

Fourth edition prepared for the Guarantors of Brain, 1999–2000

Fifth edition prepared for the Guarantors of Brain, 2009–2010

Sixth edition prepared for the Guarantors of Brain, 2020–2022

M. D. O'Brien, MD, FRCP

The Guarantors of *Brain* are very grateful to:

Patricia Archer, PhD for the drawings of the brachial plexus and lumbosacral plexus
Ralph Hutchings for the photography
Paul Richardson, Richard Tibbitts and **Joanna Cameron** for the artwork and diagrams
Michael Hutchinson, MB, BDS and **Robert Whitaker,** MA, MD, MChir, FRCS for advice on the neuroanatomy
Sarah Keer-Keer, (Harcourt Publishers) for her help and encouragement.

This atlas is intended as a guide to the examination of patients with lesions of peripheral nerves or nerve roots.

Examination should if possible be conducted in a warm and quiet room where patient and examiner will be free from distraction. Most patients will be unfamiliar with the procedures in a neurologic examination, so the nature and object of the tests should be explained in some detail to secure their interest and cooperation.

MOTOR TESTING

Inspection: Look for abnormal posture, wasting and fasciculation with the limb at rest.

Tone: In adults, the assessment of tone is only useful for upper motor neuron and extrapyramidal lesions.

Power: Muscle power is assessed by testing the strength of movement at a single joint, which is usually achieved by more than one muscle acting in different ways, and these may have different spinal root and peripheral nerve supplies.

A muscle may act as a *prime mover*, as a *fixator*, as an *antagonist*, or as a *synergist*. Thus the flexor carpi ulnaris acts as a *prime mover* when it flexes and adducts the wrist, a *fixator* when it immobilises the pisiform bone during contraction of the adductor digiti minimi, an *antagonist* when it resists extension of the wrist, and a *synergist* when the digits but not the wrists are extended.

CHOICE OF MOVEMENT

Ideally, movements should be chosen that help to differentiate upper from lower motor neuron lesions and be innervated by a single spinal root and peripheral nerve; and in peripheral nerve lesions, to identify the affected nerve and the site of the lesion. Therefore preference should be given to muscles that have a single root innervation and preferably an easily elicitable reflex, a single peripheral nerve innervation, be the main or only muscle effecting the movement, and one that can be seen and felt. This is not often possible, especially in the lower limb. The table on page 66 lists the commonly tested movements; indicates whether they are more obviously weaker in upper motor neuron lesions; and gives their principal root supply, relevant reflex if there is one, peripheral nerve, and main effector muscle.

TECHNIQUE

When testing a movement, the limb should be firmly supported proximal to the relevant joint so that the test is confined to the chosen muscle group and does not require the patient to fix the limb proximally by muscle contraction. In this book, this principle is illustrated in Figs 13, 20, 30, 33 among others. In some illustrations, the examiner's supporting hand has been omitted for clarity (e.g. Figs 32, 34–36, 50, 55). The amount of leverage applied should be such that a patient with normal strength is evenly matched with the examiner, so that minimal weakness is more easily appreciated (e.g. Figs 23, 72). However, the same technique should be used for all patients so that the examiner can acquire experience of the variability in strength of different subjects. Optimal techniques are illustrated in the figures.

Muscle power may be recorded using the Medical Research Council (MRC) scale but this is not a linear scale, and subdivisions of grade 4 are often necessary. Grades 4−, 4 and 4+ may be used to indicate movement against slight, moderate and strong resistance, respectively.

MRC SCALE FOR MUSCLE STRENGTH

0	No contraction
1	Flicker or trace of contraction
2	Full range of active movement, with gravity eliminated
3	Active movement against gravity
4	Active movement against gravity and resistance
5	Normal power

In the peripheral nerve diagrams, muscles are shown in the usual order of innervation; the origin of their motor supply from nerve trunks and the origin of the cutaneous branches are also shown, which are guides to the level of a lesion. In the figures showing methods of testing, the usual nerve supply to each muscle is stated along with the spinal segments from which they are derived, the more important of these are in bold type. Tables showing limb muscles arranged according to their supply by individual nerve roots and peripheral nerves are on pages 64 and 65.

SENSORY TESTING

Asking the patient to outline the area of sensory abnormality can be a useful guide to the detailed examination. If this clearly indicates the distribution of a peripheral nerve (e.g. the lateral cutaneous nerve of the thigh, meralgia paresthetica, Fig. 61), the area can be mapped to light touch, tested with cotton wool or a light finger touch and to pain using a clean pin (not a needle, which is designed to cut the skin). Work from the insensitive area towards an area of normal sensation. If the area of sensory abnormality is hypersensitive (hyperpathia), the direction is reversed.

Otherwise, it may be helpful to divide sensory testing into those modalities that travel in the ipsilateral posterior columns of the spinal cord (light touch, vibration and joint position sense) and those that travel in the crossed spinothalamic tracts (pain and temperature). Appreciation of vibration, a repetitive touch/pressure stimulus, is a sensitive test for demyelinating peripheral neuropathies. Two-point discrimination is a sensitive and quantifiable test of light touch, but it is only reliable on the face and fingertips. Always start with a stimulus at or below the normal threshold and coarsen the stimulus as required.

There is considerable overlap in the area of skin (dermatome) supplied by consecutive nerve roots, so that section of a single root may result in a very small area of sensory impairment. Conversely, the rash of herpes zoster may be quite extensive because it affects the whole area that has any supply from the affected root. The dermatome illustrations in Figs 90 through 97 are a compromise. The heavier axial lines, which separate nonconsecutive dermatomes, are more reliable as boundaries. The area of impairment with a peripheral nerve lesion is more reliable and consistent than that from a nerve root lesion. The areas shown in the figures are the usual ones. Some nerves show considerable variation between patients (see Figs 27, 61 and 64) and others are much more consistent (e.g. the ulnar nerve reliably splits at least part of the ring finger, see Fig. 48).

The two principal causes of a mononeuropathy are:
1. Entrapment by anatomic structures, where a nerve passes down a fibro-osseous tunnel or crosses a fascial plane
2. Compression by external forces, often where the nerve lies relatively unprotected between skin and bone

1. ENTRAPMENT NEUROPATHIES

Median nerve (page 26):
   Pronator syndrome: the nerve is trapped between the two heads of pronator teres
   Anterior interosseous nerve: the nerve may be trapped between the two heads of pronator teres with the median nerve or separately, in which case neuralgic amyotrophy is a possible diagnosis
   Carpal tunnel syndrome: the nerve is trapped in the carpal tunnel beneath the flexor retinaculum
Ulnar nerve (page 32):
   Cubital tunnel syndrome: the nerve is trapped between the two heads of flexor carpi ulnaris when the elbow is fully flexed
Posterior interosseous nerve: the nerve may be trapped between the two heads of supinator at the arcade of Frohse
Dorsal cutaneous branches of the intercostal nerves from T3 to T6 (notalgia paresthetica, page 13): the nerves are trapped as they pass through the erector spinae muscles
Lateral cutaneous nerve of the thigh (meralgia paresthetica, page 42): the nerve is trapped as it passes through the inguinal ligament medial to the anterior superior iliac spine
Common fibular nerve (page 45): the nerve is trapped at the fibular head between the insertion of fibularis longus and the fibula

2. COMPRESSION NEUROPATHIES

Radial nerve (page 18):
   'Saturday night palsy': the nerve is compressed against the shaft of the humerus
Superficial radial nerve: the nerve may be compressed against the radius at the lateral border of the forearm
Ulnar nerve (page 32):
   'Tardy ulnar palsy': the nerve is compressed in the ulnar groove
   Guyon's canal: the nerve may be compressed in Guyon's canal, usually by a ganglion
   Deep motor branch: may be compressed at the hook of the hamate
Sciatic nerve (page 50): the nerve may be compressed as it enters the thigh below gluteus maximus
Posterior cutaneous nerve of the thigh (page 43): may be compressed as it enters the thigh below gluteus maximus
Common fibular nerve (page 45): may be compressed against the head of the fibula
These sites are indicated in the figures by a red arrow.
   This section excludes obvious causes of trauma such as stab wounds, compound fractures, bullet wounds, and surgery where the site of the lesion is usually obvious. Note that a mononeuropathy may be the presenting feature of a mononeuritis multiplex, an underlying polyneuropathy, a systemic vasculitis, diabetes, or a familial liability to pressure palsies.
   For a detailed discussion of the clinical features of the mononeuropathies, see Staal A, van Gijn J, Spaans F. *Mononeuropathies, Examination, Diagnosis and Treatment.* London: WB Saunders; 1999. ISBN 0-7020-1779-5.

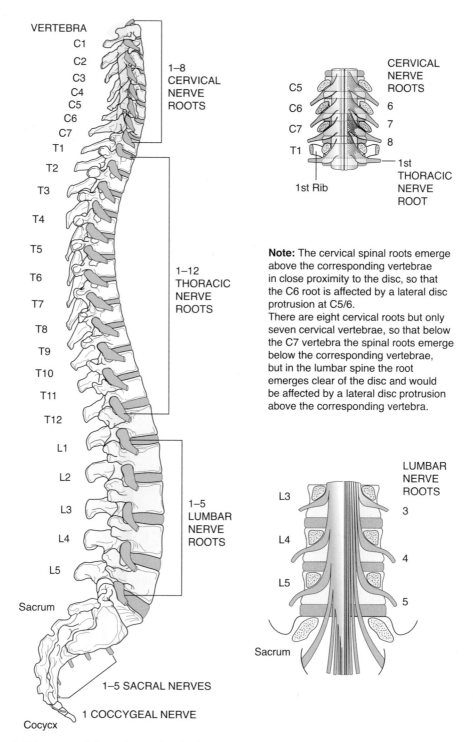

Note: The cervical spinal roots emerge above the corresponding vertebrae in close proximity to the disc, so that the C6 root is affected by a lateral disc protrusion at C5/6.

There are eight cervical roots but only seven cervical vertebrae, so that below the C7 vertebra the spinal roots emerge below the corresponding vertebrae, but in the lumbar spine the root emerges clear of the disc and would be affected by a lateral disc protrusion above the corresponding vertebra.

Fig. 1 Diagram of the spine and spinal nerve roots.

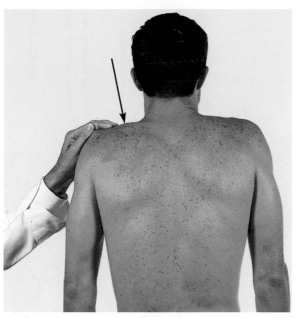

Fig. 2 Trapezius (Spinal accessory nerve and C3, C4).
The patient is elevating the shoulder against resistance.
Arrow: The thick upper part of the muscle can be seen and felt.

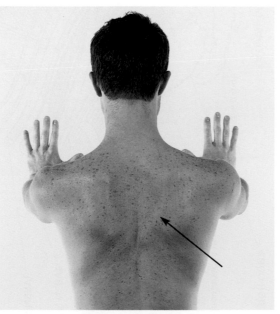

Fig. 3 Trapezius (Spinal accessory nerve and C3, C4).
The patient is pushing the palms of the hands hard against a wall with the elbows fully extended.
Arrow: The lower fibres of the trapezius can be seen and felt.

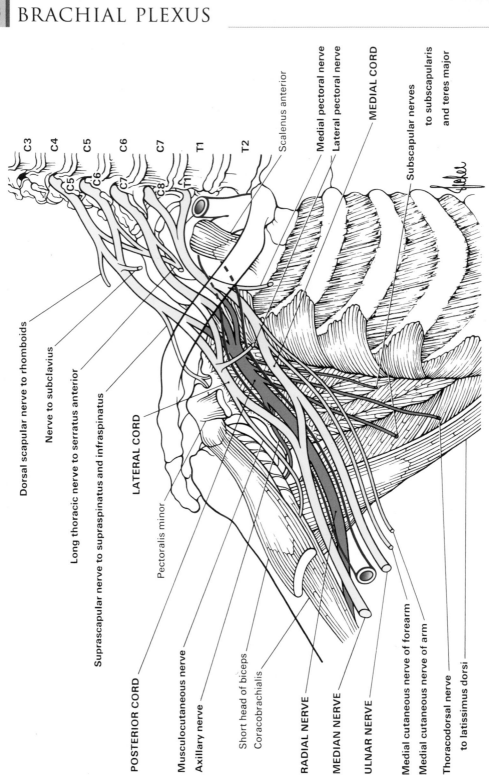

C3
C4
C5
C6
C7
T1
T2

C5
C6
C7
C8
T1

Scalenus anterior

Medial pectoral nerve
Lateral pectoral nerve

MEDIAL CORD

Subscapular nerves
to subscapularis
and teres major

Dorsal scapular nerve to rhomboids

Nerve to subclavius

Long thoracic nerve to serratus anterior

Suprascapular nerve to supraspinatus and infraspinatus

LATERAL CORD

Pectoralis minor

POSTERIOR CORD

Musculocutaneous nerve

Axillary nerve

Short head of biceps
Coracobrachialis

RADIAL NERVE

MEDIAN NERVE

ULNAR NERVE

Medial cutaneous nerve of forearm

Medial cutaneous nerve of arm

Thoracodorsal nerve
to latissimus dorsi

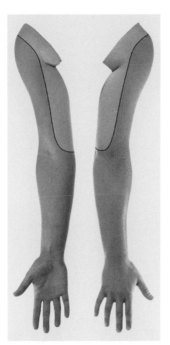

Fig. 5 The approximate area within which sensory changes may be found in complete lesions of the brachial plexus (C5, C6, C7, C8, T1).

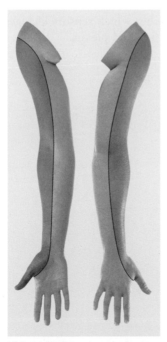

Fig. 6 The approximate area within which sensory changes may be found in lesions of the upper roots (C5, C6) of the brachial plexus.

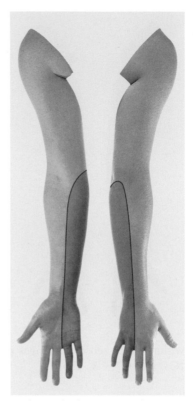

Fig. 7 The approximate area within which sensory changes may be found in lesions of the lower roots (C8, T1) of the brachial plexus.

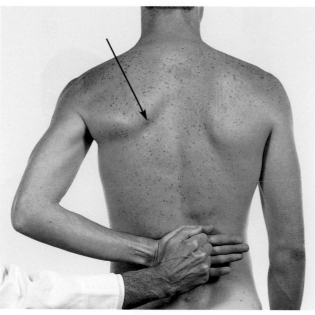

Fig. 8 Rhomboids (Dorsal scapular nerve; C4, C5).
The patient is pressing the palm of the hand backwards against the examiner's hand.
Arrow: The muscle bellies can be felt and sometimes seen.

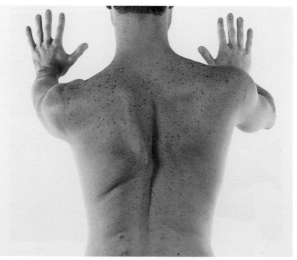

Fig. 9 Serratus Anterior (Long thoracic nerve; C5, **C6**, C7).
The patient is pushing against a wall. The left serratus anterior is weak and there is winging of the scapula.

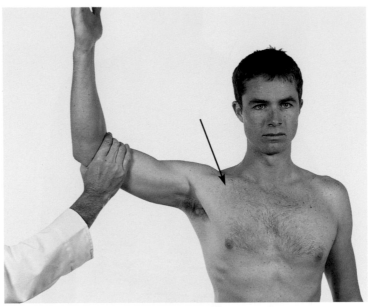

Fig. 10 Pectoralis Major: Clavicular head (Lateral pectoral nerve; C5, C6).
The upper arm is above the horizontal and the patient is pushing forward against the examiner's hand.
Arrow: The clavicular head of the pectoralis major can be seen and felt.

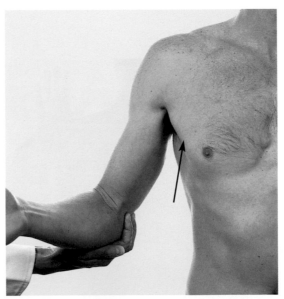

Fig. 11 Pectoralis Major: Sternocostal head (Lateral and medial pectoral nerves; C6, C7, C8, T1).
The patient is adducting the upper arm against resistance.
Arrow: The sternocostal head can be seen and felt.

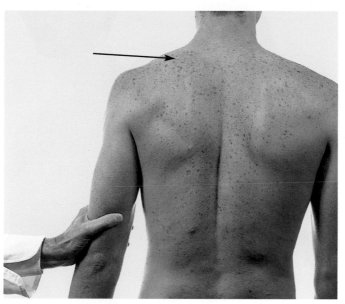

Fig. 12 Supraspinatus (Suprascapular nerve; C5, C6).
The patient is abducting the upper arm against resistance.
Arrow: The muscle belly can be felt and sometimes seen.

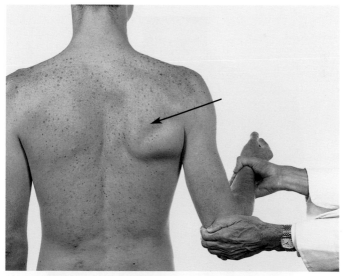

Fig. 13 Infraspinatus (Suprascapular nerve; C5, C6).
The patient is externally rotating the upper arm at the shoulder against resistance. The examiner's right hand is resisting the movement and supporting the forearm with the elbow at a right angle; the examiner's left hand is supporting the elbow and preventing abduction of the arm.
Arrow: The muscle belly can be seen and felt.

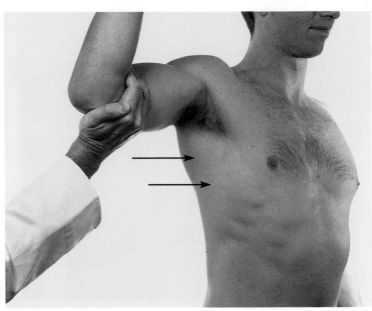

Fig. 14 Latissimus Dorsi (Thoracodorsal nerve; C6, **C7**, C8).
The upper arm is horizontal and the patient is adducting it against resistance.
Lower arrow: The muscle belly can be seen and felt. *Upper arrow:* Indicates teres major.

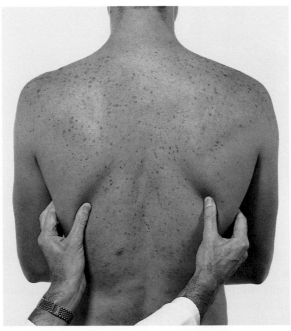

Fig. 15 Latissimus Dorsi (Thoracodorsal nerve; C6, **C7**, C8).
The muscle bellies can be felt to contract when the patient coughs.

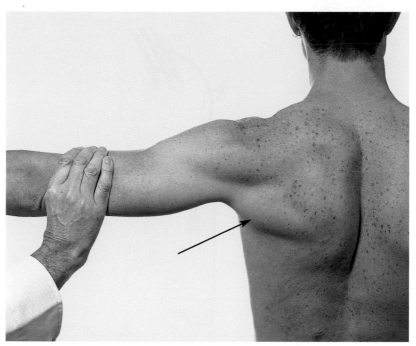

Fig. 16 Teres Major (Subscapular nerve; C5, C6, C7).
The patient is adducting the elevated upper arm against resistance.
Arrow: The muscle belly can be seen and felt.

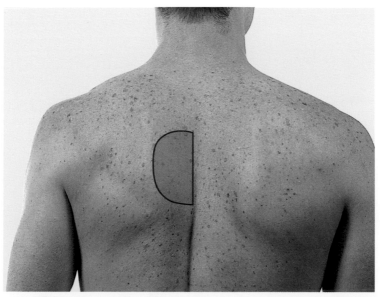

Fig. 17 The approximate area within which sensory changes may be found in lesions of the posterior cutaneous branches of the intercostal nerves from T2 to T6 (notalgia paresthetica).

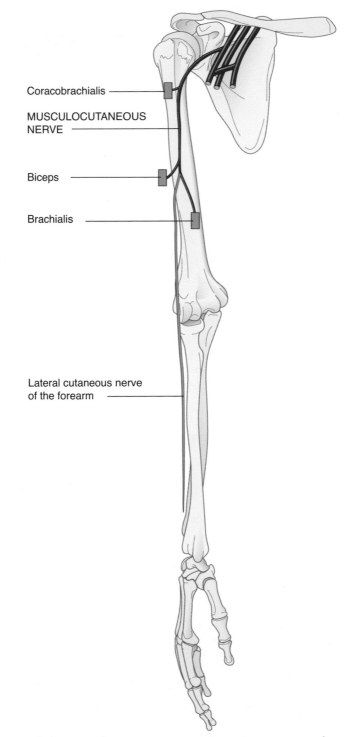

Coracobrachialis

MUSCULOCUTANEOUS
NERVE

Biceps

Brachialis

Lateral cutaneous nerve
of the forearm

Fig. 18 Diagram of the musculocutaneous nerve, its major cutaneous branch and the muscles it supplies.

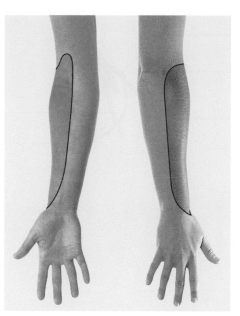

Fig. 19 The approximate area within which sensory changes may be found in lesions of the musculocutaneous nerve. (The distribution of the lateral cutaneous nerve of the forearm.)

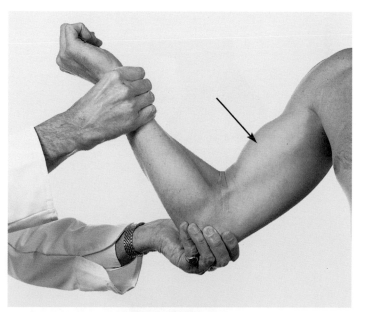

Fig. 20 Biceps (Musculocutaneous nerve; **C5, C6**). The patient is flexing the supinated forearm against resistance. *Arrow:* The muscle belly can be seen and felt.

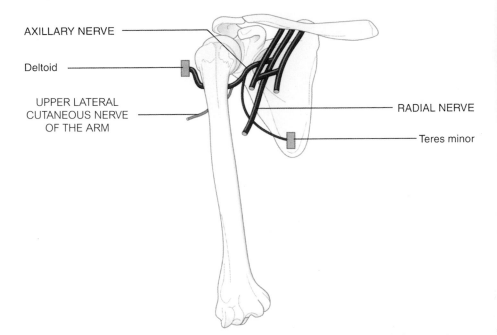

AXILLARY NERVE

Deltoid

UPPER LATERAL
CUTANEOUS NERVE
OF THE ARM

RADIAL NERVE

Teres minor

Fig. 21 Diagram of the axillary nerve, its major cutaneous branch and the muscles it supplies.

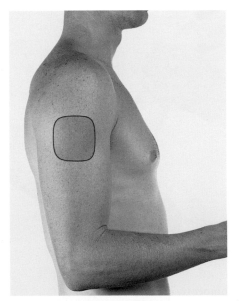

Fig. 22 The approximate area within which sensory changes may be found in lesions of the axillary nerve.

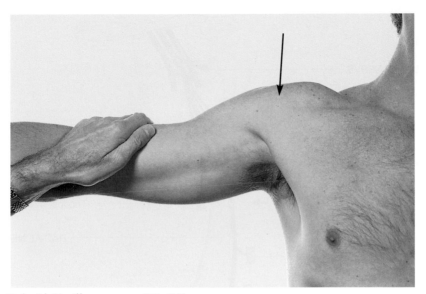

Fig. 23 Deltoid (Axillary nerve; C5, C6).
The patient is abducting the upper arm against resistance.
Arrow: The anterior and middle fibres of the muscle can be seen and felt.

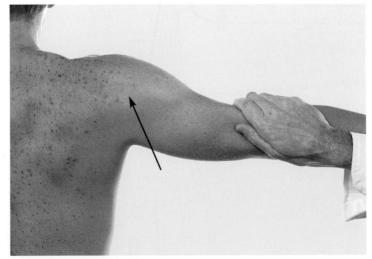

Fig. 24 Deltoid (Axillary nerve; C5, C6).
The patient is retracting the abducted upper arm against resistance.
Arrow: The posterior fibres of the deltoid can be seen and felt.

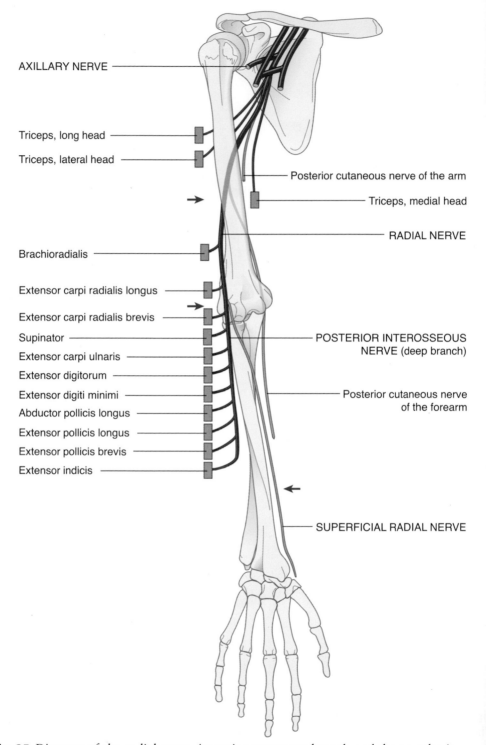

AXILLARY NERVE

Triceps, long head

Triceps, lateral head

Posterior cutaneous nerve of the arm

Triceps, medial head

RADIAL NERVE

Brachioradialis

Extensor carpi radialis longus

Extensor carpi radialis brevis

Supinator

POSTERIOR INTEROSSEOUS
NERVE (deep branch)

Extensor carpi ulnaris

Extensor digitorum

Extensor digiti minimi

Posterior cutaneous nerve
of the forearm

Abductor pollicis longus

Extensor pollicis longus

Extensor pollicis brevis

Extensor indicis

SUPERFICIAL RADIAL NERVE

Fig. 25 Diagram of the radial nerve, its major cutaneous branch and the muscles it supplies.

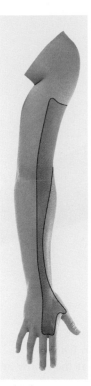

Fig. 26 The approximate area within which sensory changes may be found in high lesions of the radial nerve (above the origin of lower lateral cutaneous nerve of the arm and the posterior cutaneous nerves of the arm and forearm). The average area is usually considerably smaller and absence of sensory changes has been recorded.

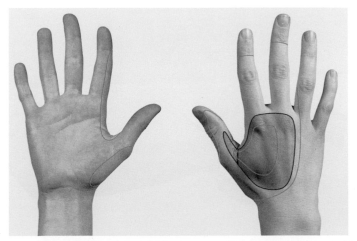

Fig. 27 The approximate area within which sensory changes may be found in lesions of the radial nerve above the elbow joint and below the origin of the posterior cutaneous nerve of the forearm (the distribution of the superficial terminal branch of the radial nerve). Usual area shaded with *dark blue line*; *light blue lines* show small and large areas.

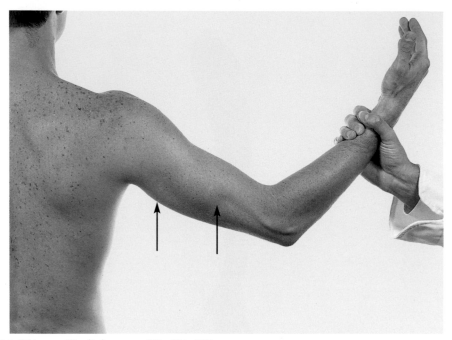

Fig. 28 Triceps (Radial nerve; C6, **C7**, C8).
The patient is extending the forearm at the elbow against resistance.
Arrows: The long and lateral heads of the muscle can be seen and felt.

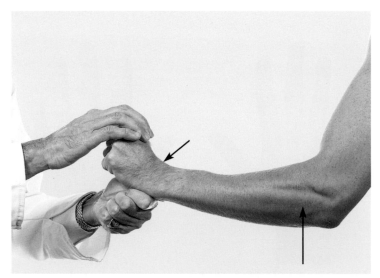

Fig. 29 Extensor Carpi Radialis Longus (Radial nerve; C5, **C6**).
The patient is extending and abducting the hand at the wrist against resistance.
Arrows: The muscle belly and tendon can be felt and usually seen.

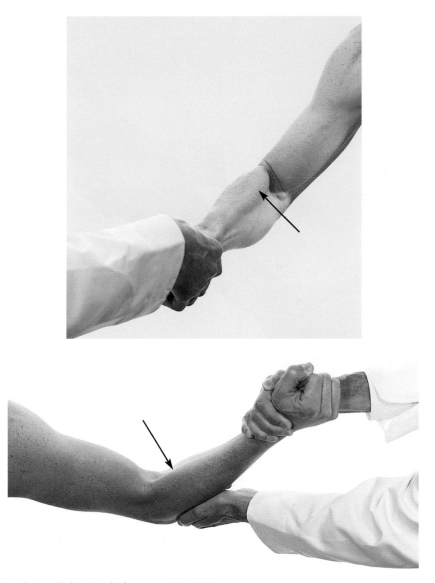

Fig. 30 Brachioradialis (Radial nerve; C5, C6).
The patient is flexing the forearm against resistance with the forearm midway between
pronation and supination.
Arrows: The muscle belly can be seen and felt.

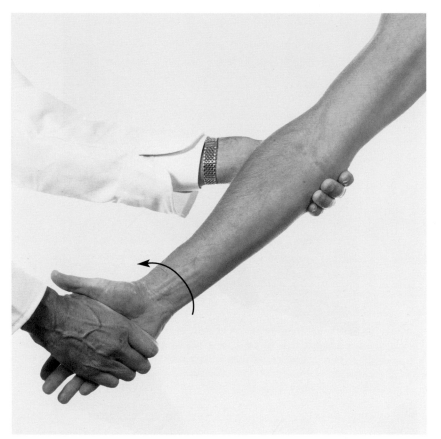

Fig. 31 Supinator (Radial nerve; C6, C7).
The patient is supinating the forearm against resistance with the forearm extended at the elbow.

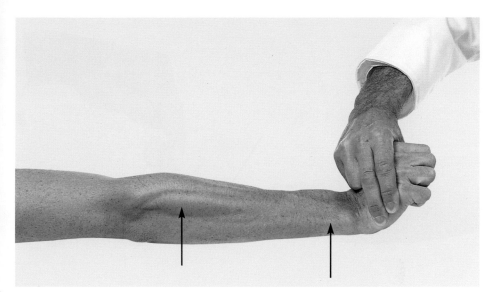

Fig. 32 Extensor Carpi Ulnaris (Posterior interosseous nerve; C7, C8).
The patient is extending and adducting the hand at the wrist against resistance.
Arrows: The muscle belly and the tendon can be seen and felt.

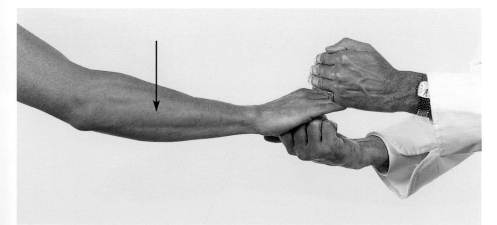

Fig. 33 Extensor Digitorum (Posterior interosseous nerve; C7, C8).
The patient's hand is firmly supported by the examiner's right hand. Extension at the metacarpophalangeal joints is maintained against the resistance of the fingers of the examiner's left hand.
Arrow: The muscle belly can be seen and felt.

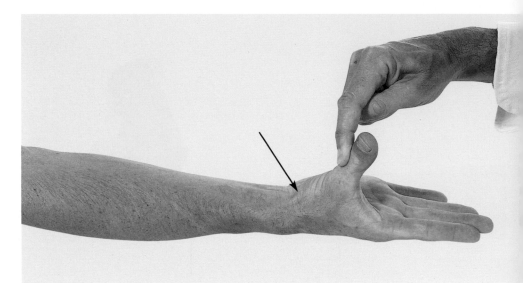

Fig. 34 Abductor Pollicis Longus (Posterior interosseous nerve; **C7**, C8).
The patient is abducting the thumb at the carpometacarpal joint in a plane at right angles to the palm.
Arrow: The tendon can be seen and felt anterior and closely adjacent to the tendon of extensor pollicis brevis (see Fig. 36).

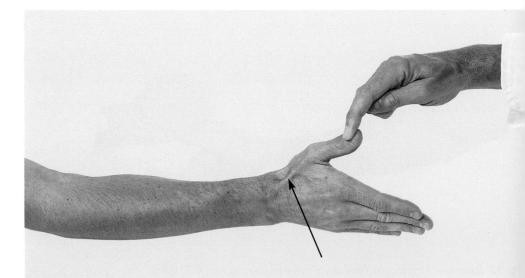

Fig. 35 Extensor Pollicis Longus (Posterior interosseous nerve; **C7**, C8).
The patient is extending the thumb at the interphalangeal joint against resistance.
Arrow: The tendon can be seen and felt.

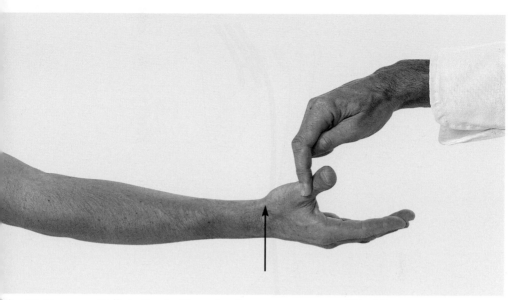

Fig. 36 Extensor Pollicis Brevis (Posterior interosseous nerve; C7, C8).
The patient is extending the thumb at the metacarpophalangeal joint against resistance.
Arrow: The tendon can be seen and felt (see Fig. 34).

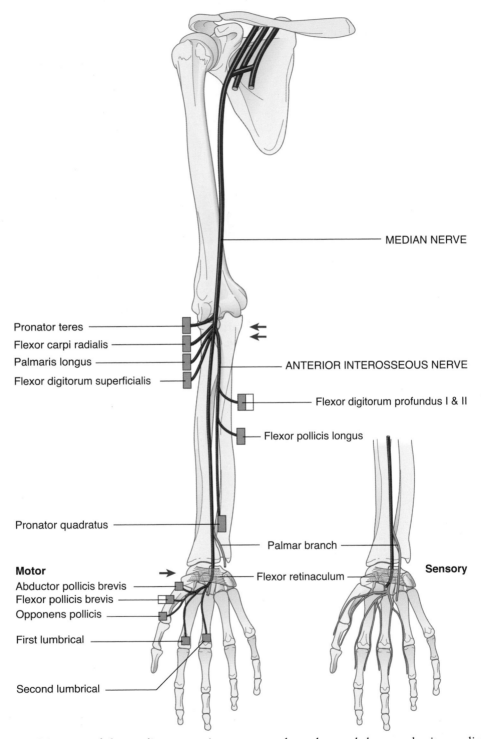

Fig. 37 Diagram of the median nerve, its cutaneous branches and the muscles it supplies. Note: The white rectangle signifies that the muscle indicated receives a part of its nerve supply from another peripheral nerve (see Figs 47, 59 and 60).

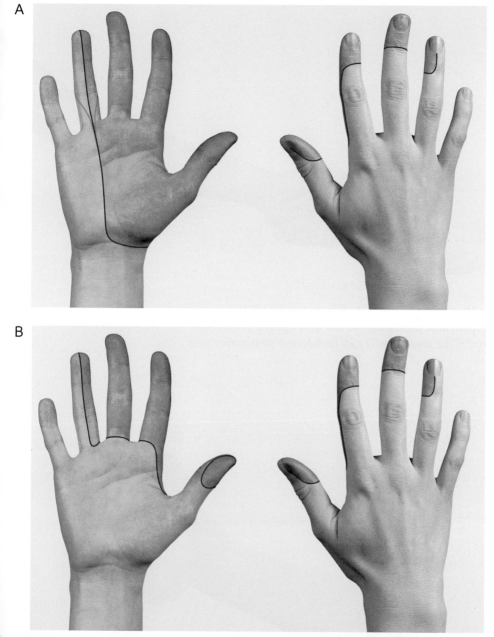

Fig. 38 The approximate areas within which sensory changes may be found in lesions of the median nerve in: **A** the forearm, **B** the carpal tunnel. Note sparing of the palmar branch, which does not go through the carpal tunnel.

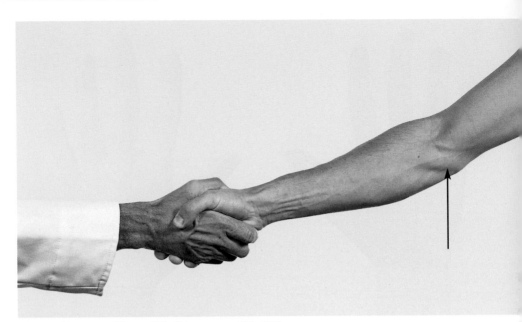

Fig. 39 Pronator Teres (Median nerve; C6, **C7**).
The patient is pronating the forearm against resistance.
Arrow: The muscle belly can be felt and sometimes seen.

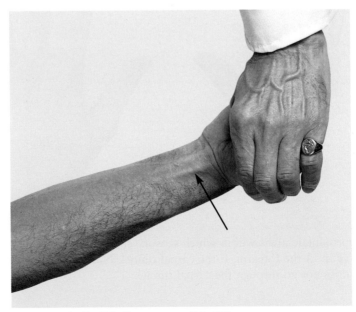

Fig. 40 Flexor Carpi Radialis (Median nerve; C6, C7).
The patient is flexing and abducting the hand at the wrist against resistance.
Arrow: The tendon can be seen and felt.

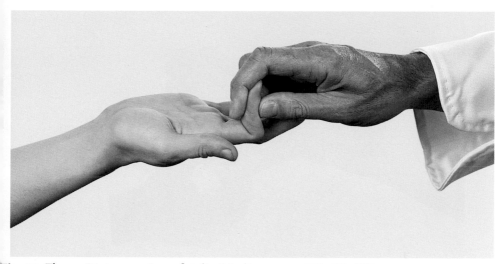

Fig. 41 Flexor Digitorum Superficialis (Median nerve; C7, **C8**, T1).
The patient is flexing the finger at the proximal interphalangeal joint against resistance with the proximal phalanx fixed. This test does not eliminate the possibility of flexion at the proximal interphalangeal joint being produced by flexor digitorum profundus.

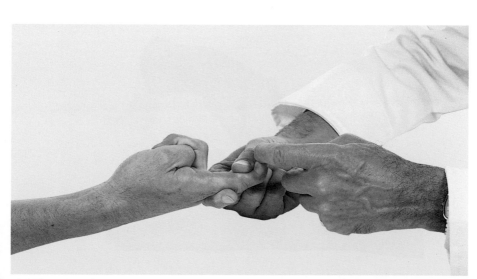

Fig. 42 Flexor Digitorum Profundus I and II (Anterior interosseous nerve; C7, C8).
The patient is flexing the distal phalanx of the index finger against resistance with the middle phalanx fixed.

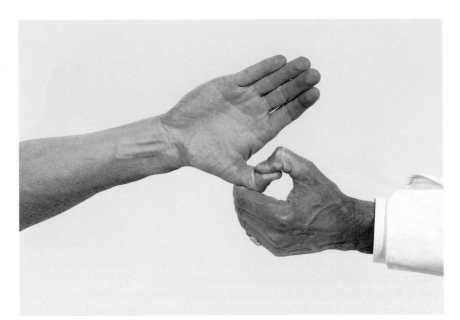

Fig. 43 Flexor Pollicis Longus (Anterior interosseous nerve; C7, **C8**).
The patient is flexing the distal phalanx of the thumb against resistance while the proximal phalanx is fixed.

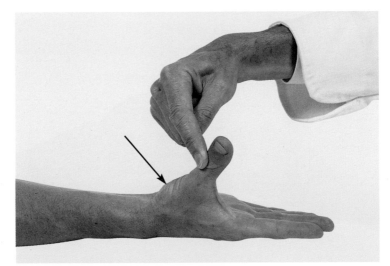

Fig. 44 Abductor Pollicis Brevis (Median nerve; C8, **T1**).
The patient is abducting the thumb at right angles to the palm against resistance.
Arrow: The muscle can be seen and felt.

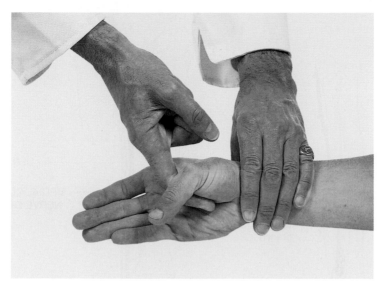

Fig. 45 Opponens Pollicis (Median nerve; C8, **T1**).
The patient is touching the base of the little finger with the thumb against resistance.

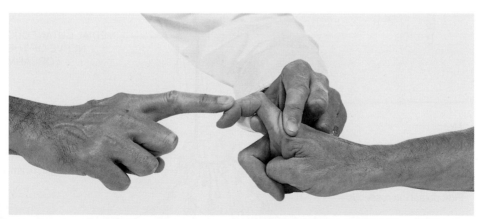

Fig. 46 First Lumbrical-Interosseous Muscle (Median and ulnar nerves; C8, **T1**).
The patient is extending the finger at the proximal interphalangeal joint against resistance with the metacarpophalangeal joint hyperextended and fixed.

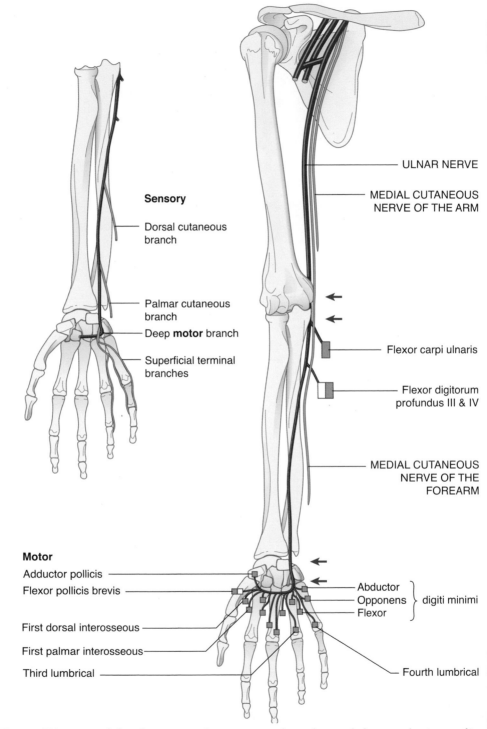

Sensory

Dorsal cutaneous branch

Palmar cutaneous branch

Deep **motor** branch

Superficial terminal branches

ULNAR NERVE

MEDIAL CUTANEOUS NERVE OF THE ARM

Flexor carpi ulnaris

Flexor digitorum profundus III & IV

MEDIAL CUTANEOUS NERVE OF THE FOREARM

Motor

Adductor pollicis

Flexor pollicis brevis

First dorsal interosseous

First palmar interosseous

Third lumbrical

Abductor
Opponens } digiti minimi
Flexor

Fourth lumbrical

Fig. 47 Diagram of the ulnar nerve, its cutaneous branches and the muscles it supplies.

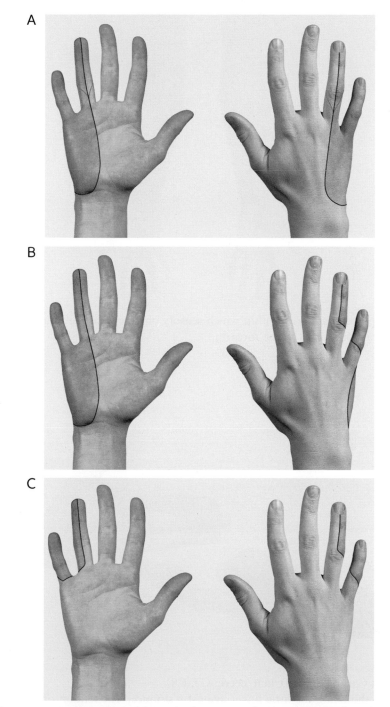

Fig. 48 The approximate areas within which sensory changes may be found in lesions of the ulnar nerve: **A** above the origin of the dorsal cutaneous branch, **B** below the origin of the dorsal cutaneous branch and above the origin of the palmar branch, **C** below the origin of the palmar branch.

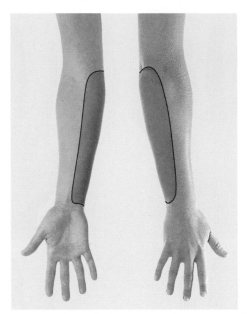

Fig. 49 The approximate area within which sensory changes may be found in lesions of the medial cutaneous nerve of the forearm.

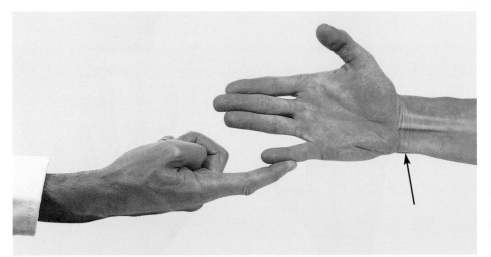

Fig. 50 Flexor Carpi Ulnaris (Ulnar nerve; C7, C8).
The patient is abducting the little finger against resistance. The tendon of flexor carpi ulnaris can be seen and felt *(arrow)* as the muscle comes into action to fix the pisiform bone from which abductor digiti minimi arises. If flexor carpi ulnaris is intact, the tendon is seen even when abductor digiti minimi is paralysed (see also Fig. 51).

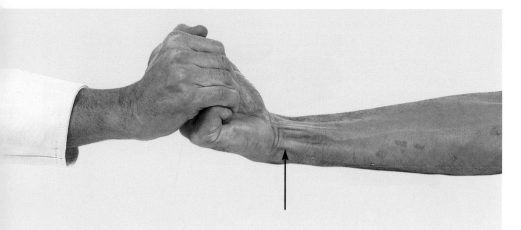

Fig. 51 Flexor Carpi Ulnaris (Ulnar nerve; **C7, C8**).
The patient is flexing and adducting the hand at the wrist against resistance.
Arrow: The tendon can be seen and felt.

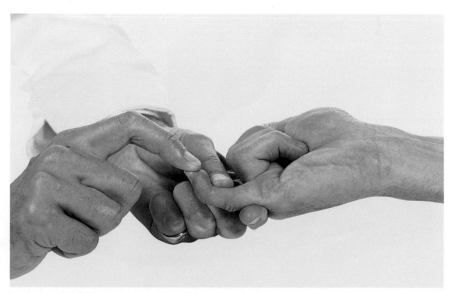

Fig. 52 Flexor Digitorum Profundus III and IV (Ulnar nerve; **C7, C8**).
The patient is flexing the distal interphalangeal joint against resistance while the middle phalanx is fixed.

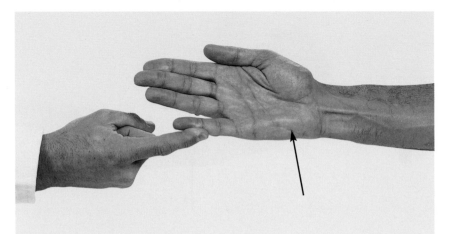

Fig. 53 Abductor Digiti Minimi (Ulnar nerve; C8, **T1**)
The patient is abducting the little finger against resistance.
Arrow: The muscle belly can be felt and seen.

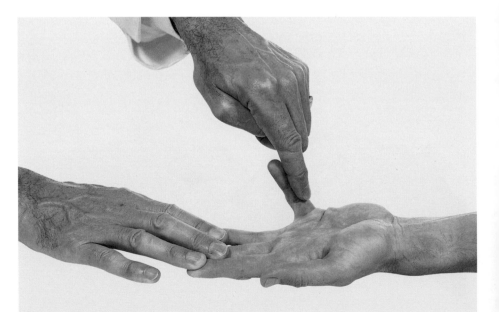

Fig. 54 Flexor Digiti Minimi (Ulnar nerve; C8, **T1**).
The patient is flexing the little finger at the metacarpophalangeal joint against resistance
with the finger extended at both interphalangeal joints.

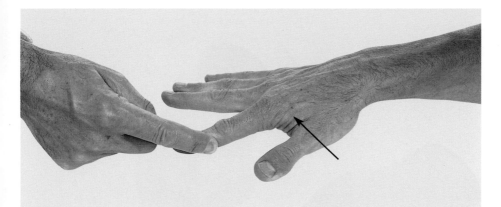

Fig. 55 First Dorsal Interosseous Muscle (Ulnar nerve; C8, **T1**).
The patient is abducting the index finger against resistance.
Arrow: The muscle belly can be felt and seen.

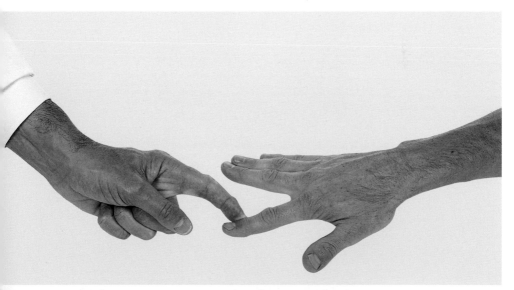

Fig. 56 Second Palmar Interosseous Muscle (Ulnar nerve; C8, **T1**).
The patient is adducting the index finger against resistance.

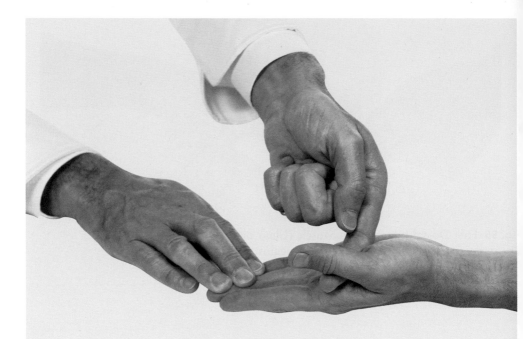

Fig. 57 Adductor Pollicis (Ulnar nerve; C8, T1).
The patient is adducting the thumb at right angles to the palm against the resistance of the examiner's finger.

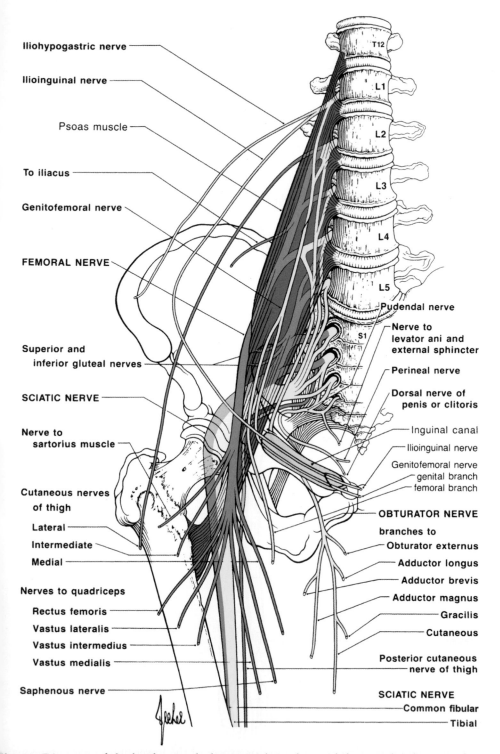

Iliohypogastric nerve

Ilioinguinal nerve

Psoas muscle

To iliacus

Genitofemoral nerve

FEMORAL NERVE

Superior and
inferior gluteal nerves

SCIATIC NERVE

Nerve to
sartorius muscle

Cutaneous nerves
of thigh

Lateral

Intermediate

Medial

Nerves to quadriceps

Rectus femoris

Vastus lateralis

Vastus intermedius

Vastus medialis

Saphenous nerve

T12

L1

L2

L3

L4

L5

S1

Pudendal nerve

Nerve to
levator ani and
external sphincter

Perineal nerve

Dorsal nerve of
penis or clitoris

Inguinal canal

Ilioinguinal nerve

Genitofemoral nerve
genital branch
femoral branch

OBTURATOR NERVE

branches to

Obturator externus

Adductor longus

Adductor brevis

Adductor magnus

Gracilis

Cutaneous

Posterior cutaneous
nerve of thigh

SCIATIC NERVE

Common fibular

Tibial

Fig. 58 Diagram of the lumbosacral plexus, its branches and the muscles they supply.

NERVES OF THE LOWER LIMB

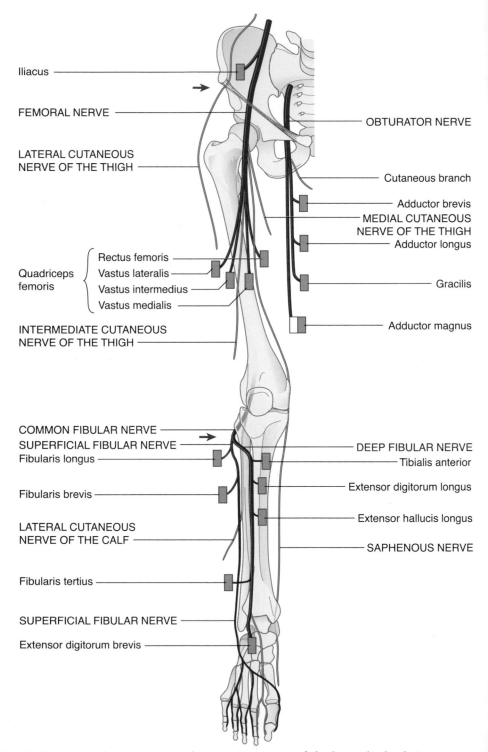

Iliacus

FEMORAL NERVE

LATERAL CUTANEOUS
NERVE OF THE THIGH

OBTURATOR NERVE

Cutaneous branch

Adductor brevis
MEDIAL CUTANEOUS
NERVE OF THE THIGH
Adductor longus

Quadriceps femoris
- Rectus femoris
- Vastus lateralis
- Vastus intermedius
- Vastus medialis

Gracilis

Adductor magnus

INTERMEDIATE CUTANEOUS
NERVE OF THE THIGH

COMMON FIBULAR NERVE
SUPERFICIAL FIBULAR NERVE
Fibularis longus

DEEP FIBULAR NERVE
Tibialis anterior

Extensor digitorum longus

Fibularis brevis

Extensor hallucis longus

LATERAL CUTANEOUS
NERVE OF THE CALF

SAPHENOUS NERVE

Fibularis tertius

SUPERFICIAL FIBULAR NERVE

Extensor digitorum brevis

Fig. 59 Diagram of the nerves on the anterior aspect of the lower limb, their cutaneous branches and the muscles they supply.

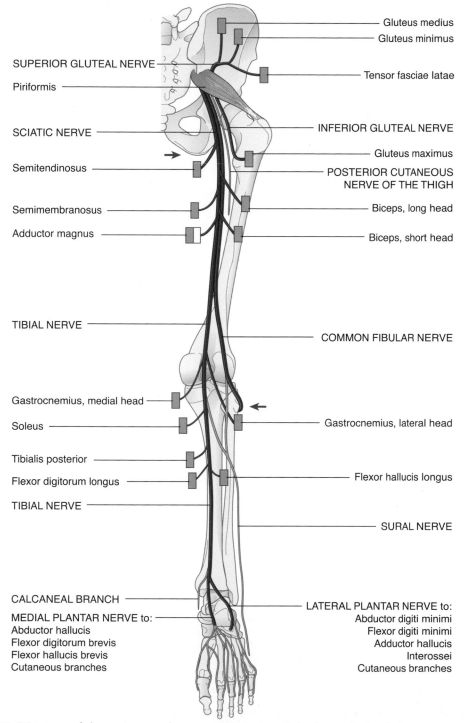

SUPERIOR GLUTEAL NERVE

Piriformis

SCIATIC NERVE

Semitendinosus

Semimembranosus

Adductor magnus

TIBIAL NERVE

Gastrocnemius, medial head

Soleus

Tibialis posterior

Flexor digitorum longus

TIBIAL NERVE

CALCANEAL BRANCH

MEDIAL PLANTAR NERVE to:
Abductor hallucis
Flexor digitorum brevis
Flexor hallucis brevis
Cutaneous branches

Gluteus medius
Gluteus minimus

Tensor fasciae latae

INFERIOR GLUTEAL NERVE

Gluteus maximus
POSTERIOR CUTANEOUS
NERVE OF THE THIGH

Biceps, long head

Biceps, short head

COMMON FIBULAR NERVE

Gastrocnemius, lateral head

Flexor hallucis longus

SURAL NERVE

LATERAL PLANTAR NERVE to:
Abductor digiti minimi
Flexor digiti minimi
Adductor hallucis
Interossei
Cutaneous branches

Fig. 60 Diagram of the nerves on the posterior aspect of the lower limb, their cutaneous branches and the muscles they supply. Note: The tibial nerve and the common fibular nerve are separate bundles up to the piriformis.

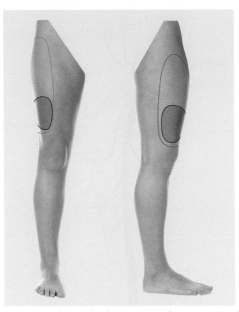

Fig. 61 The approximate area within which sensory changes may be found in lesions of the lateral cutaneous nerve of the thigh (meralgia paresthetica).
Usual area shaded with dark blue line; large area indicated with light blue line.

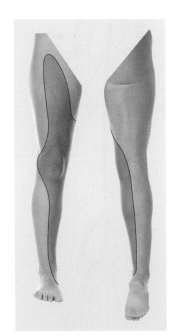

Fig. 62 The approximate area within which sensory changes may be found in lesions of the femoral nerve (the distribution of the intermediate and medial cutaneous nerves of the thigh and the saphenous nerve).

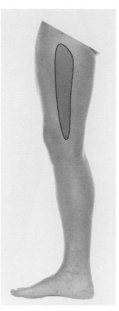

Fig. 63 The approximate area within which sensory changes may be found in lesions of the obturator nerve.

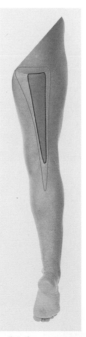

Fig. 64 The approximate area within which sensory changes may be found in lesions of the posterior cutaneous nerve of the thigh. Usual area shaded with dark blue line; large area indicated with light blue line.

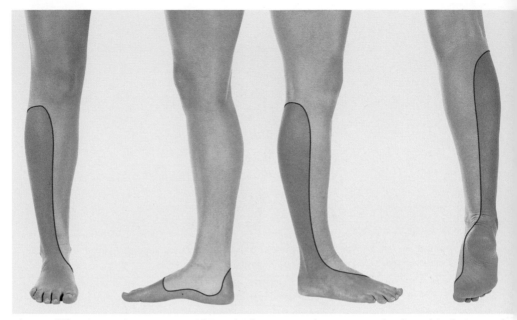

Fig. 65 The approximate area within which sensory changes may be found in lesions of the trunk of the sciatic nerve.

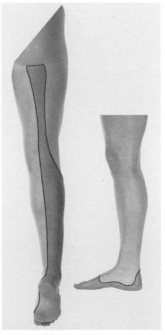

Fig. 66 The approximate area within which sensory changes may be found in lesions of both the sciatic and the posterior cutaneous nerve of the thigh.

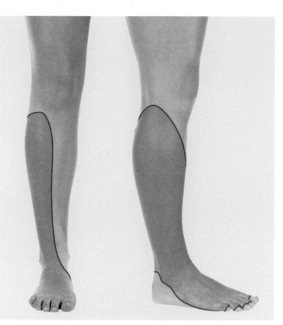

Fig. 67 The approximate area within which sensory changes may be found in lesions of the common fibular nerve above the origin of the superficial fibular nerve.

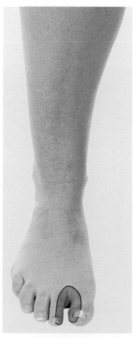

Fig. 68 The approximate area within which sensory changes may be found in lesions of the deep fibular nerve.

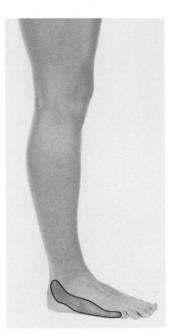

Fig. 69 The approximate area within which sensory changes may be found in lesions of the sural nerve.

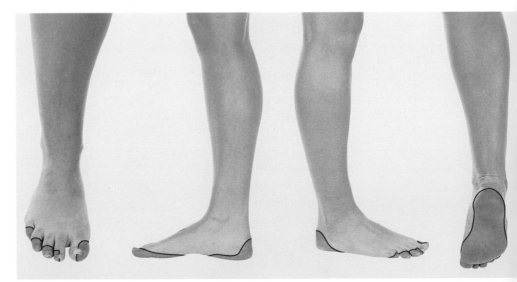

Fig. 70 The approximate area within which sensory changes may be found in lesions of the tibial nerve.

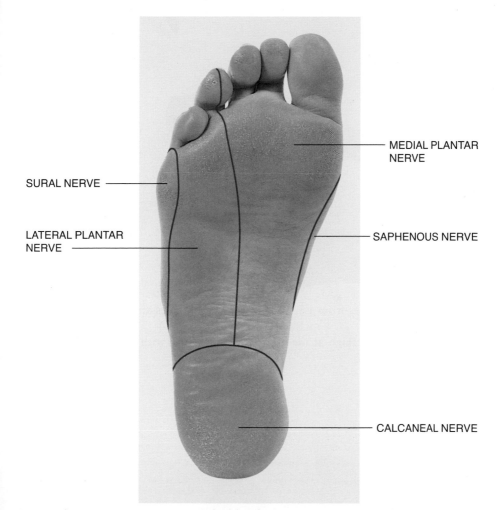

Fig. 71 The approximate areas supplied by the cutaneous nerves to the sole of the foot.

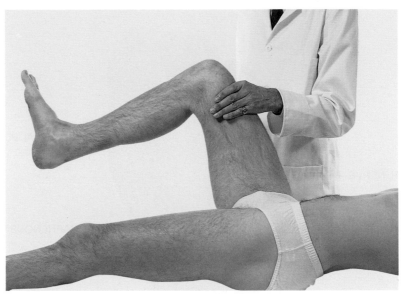

Fig. 72 Iliopsoas (branches from L1, L2 and L3 spinal nerves and femoral nerve; **L1, L2, L3**).
The patient is flexing the thigh at the hip against resistance with the leg flexed at the knee and hip.

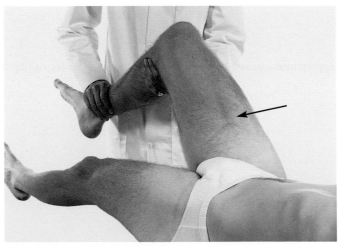

Fig. 73 Quadriceps Femoris (Femoral nerve; **L2, L3, L4**).
The patient is extending the leg against resistance with the limb flexed at the hip and knee. To detect slight weakness, the leg should be fully flexed at the knee.
Arrow: The muscle belly of rectus femoris can be seen and felt.

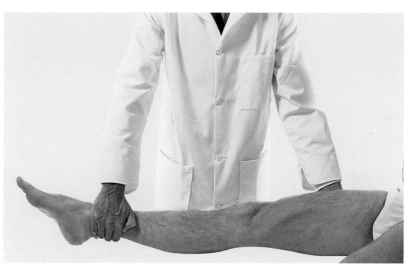

Fig. 74 Adductors (Obturator nerve; **L2, L3,** L4).
The patient lies on the back with the leg extended at the knee and is adducting the limb against resistance. The muscle bellies can be felt.

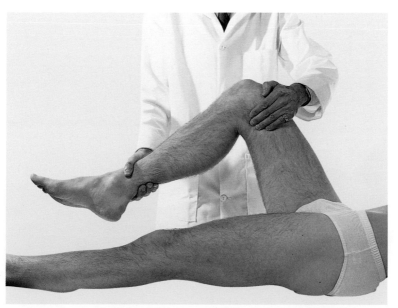

Fig. 75 Gluteus Medius and Minimus (Superior gluteal nerve; **L4, L5,** S1).
The patient lies on the back and is internally rotating the thigh against resistance with the limb flexed at the hip and knee.

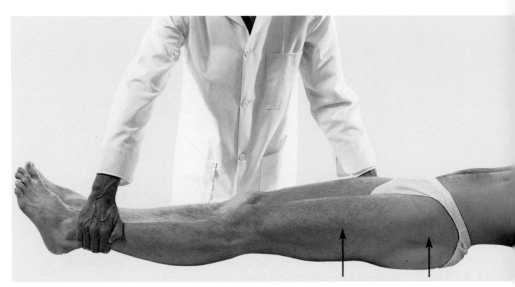

Fig. 76 Gluteus Medius and Minimus and Tensor Fasciae Latae (Superior gluteal nerve; L4, L5, S1).
The patient lies on the back with the leg extended and is abducting the limb against resistance.
Arrows: The muscle bellies can be felt and sometimes seen.

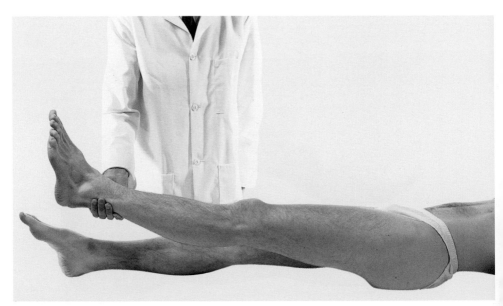

Fig. 77 Gluteus Maximus (Inferior gluteal nerve; L5, S1, S2).
The patient lies on the back with the leg extended at the knee and is extending the limb at the hip against resistance.

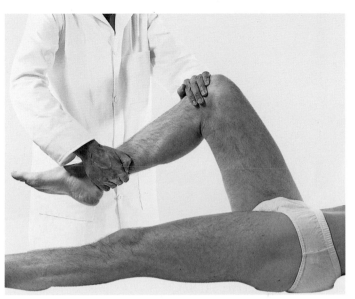

Fig. 78 Hamstring Muscles (Sciatic nerve; semitendinosus, semimembranosus and biceps; L5, S1, S2).
The patient lies on the back with the limb flexed at the hip and knee and is flexing the leg at the knee against resistance.

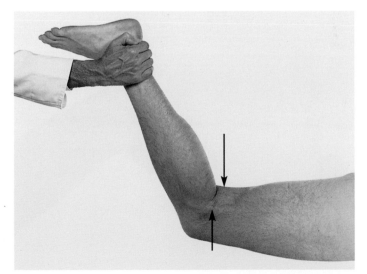

Fig. 79 Hamstring Muscles (Sciatic nerve; semitendinosus, semimembranosus and biceps; L5, S1, S2).
The patient lies face down and is flexing the leg at the knee against resistance.
Arrows: The tendons of the biceps (laterally) and semitendinosus (medially) can be felt and seen.

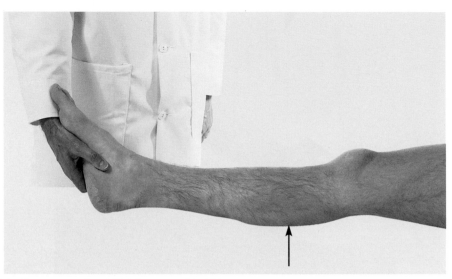

Fig. 80 Gastrocnemius (Tibial nerve; S1, S2).
The patient lies on the back with the leg extended and is plantar-flexing the foot against resistance.
Arrow: The muscle bellies can be seen and felt. To detect slight weakness, the patient should be asked to stand on one foot, raise the heel from the ground and maintain this position.

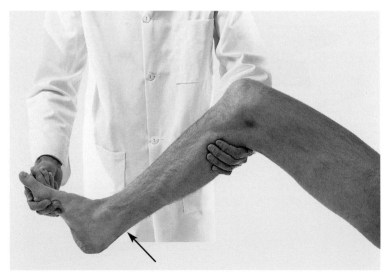

Fig. 81 Soleus (Tibial nerve; S1, S2).
The patient lies on the back with the limb flexed at the hip and knee and is plantar-flexing the foot against resistance. The muscle belly can be felt and sometimes seen below the tendon insertion of gastrocnemius.
Arrow: The Achilles tendon.

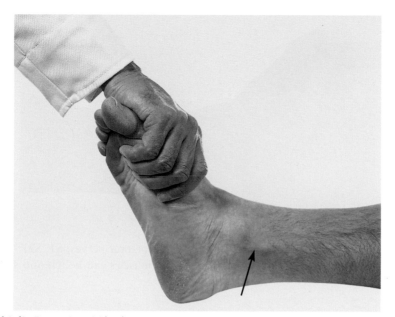

Fig. 82 Tibialis Posterior (Tibial nerve; L4, L5).
The patient is inverting the foot against resistance.
Arrow: The tendon can be seen and felt.

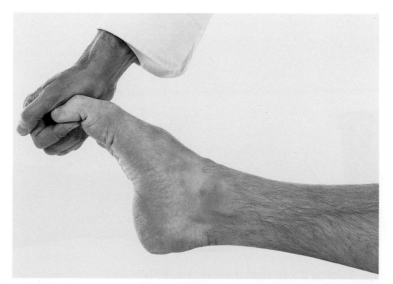

Fig. 83 Flexor Digitorum Longus, Flexor Hallucis Longus (Tibial nerve; L5, S1, S2).
The patient is flexing the toes against resistance.

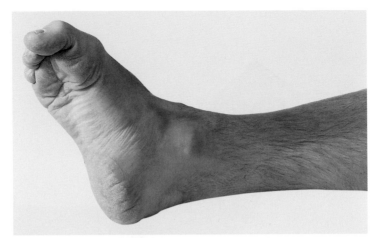

Fig. 84 Small muscles of the foot (Medial and lateral plantar nerves; S1, S2).
The patient is cupping the sole of the foot; the small muscles can be felt and sometimes seen.

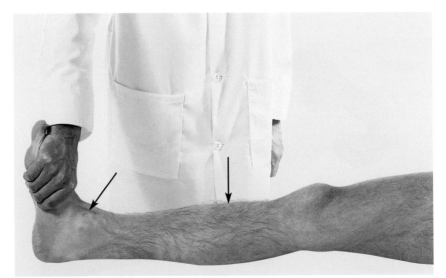

Fig. 85 Tibialis Anterior (Deep fibular nerve; L4, L5).
The patient is dorsiflexing the foot against resistance.
Arrows: The muscle belly and its tendon can be seen and felt.

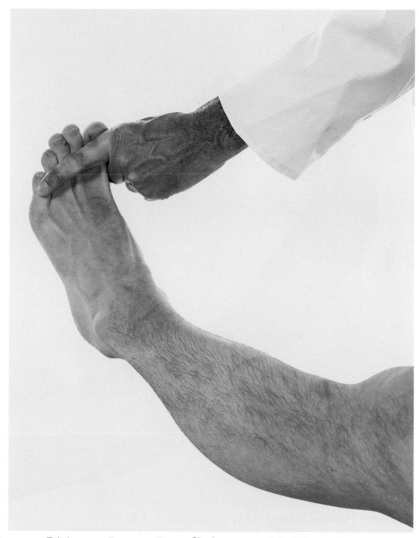

Fig. 86 Extensor Digitorum Longus (Deep fibular nerve; L5, S1).
The patient is dorsiflexing the toes against resistance. The tendons passing to the lateral four toes can be seen and felt.

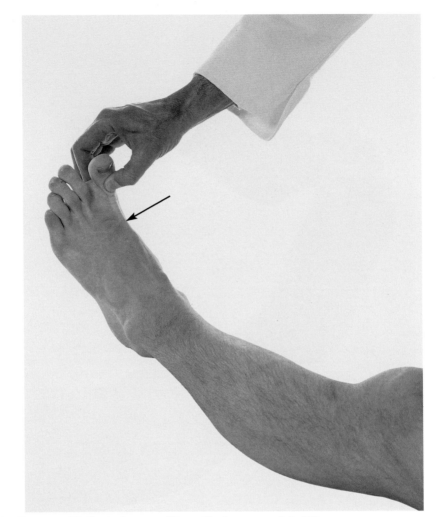

Fig. 87 Extensor Hallucis Longus (Deep fibular nerve; L5, S1).
The patient is dorsiflexing the distal phalanx of the big toe against resistance.
Arrow: The tendon can be seen and felt.

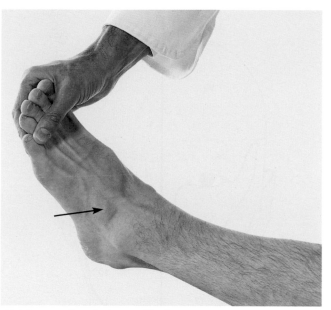

Fig. 88 Extensor Digitorum Brevis (Deep fibular nerve; L5, S1).
The patient is dorsiflexing the proximal phalanges of the toes against resistance.
Arrow: The muscle belly can be felt and sometimes seen.

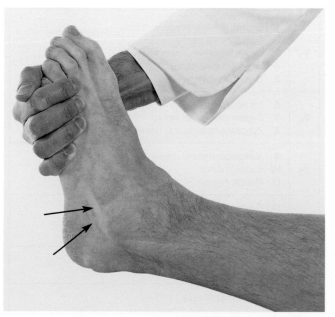

Fig. 89 Fibularis Longus and Brevis (Superficial fibular nerve; L5, S1).
The patient is everting the foot against resistance.
Upper arrow: The tendon of fibularis brevis. *Lower arrow:* The tendon of fibularis longus.

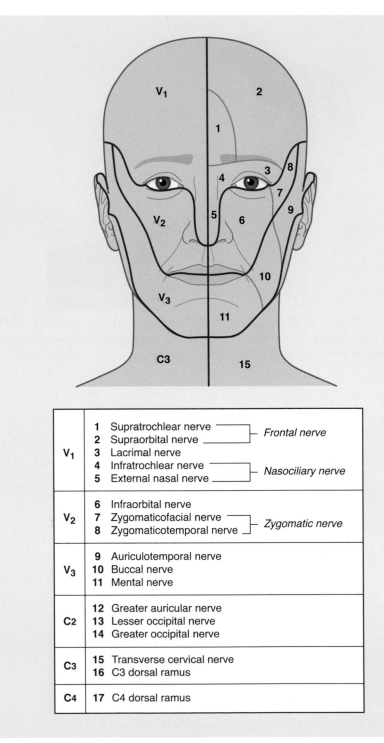

	1 Supratrochlear nerve	Frontal nerve
V₁	2 Supraorbital nerve	
	3 Lacrimal nerve	
	4 Infratrochlear nerve	Nasociliary nerve
	5 External nasal nerve	
V₂	6 Infraorbital nerve	
	7 Zygomaticofacial nerve	Zygomatic nerve
	8 Zygomaticotemporal nerve	
V₃	9 Auriculotemporal nerve	
	10 Buccal nerve	
	11 Mental nerve	
C2	12 Greater auricular nerve	
	13 Lesser occipital nerve	
	14 Greater occipital nerve	
C3	15 Transverse cervical nerve	
	16 C3 dorsal ramus	
C4	17 C4 dorsal ramus	

Figs 90, 91, 92 The approximate areas within which sensory changes may be found in lesions of the trigeminal nerve, its branches and the upper cervical nerves.

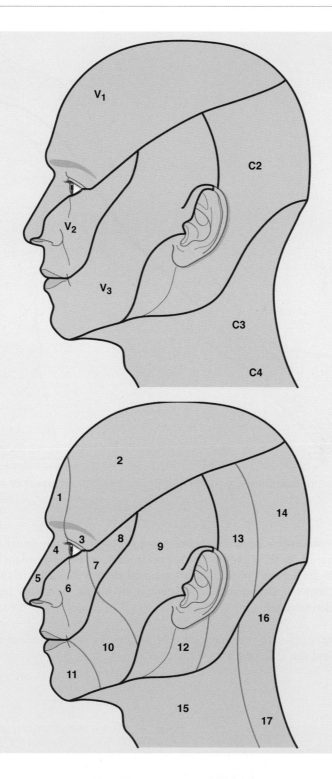

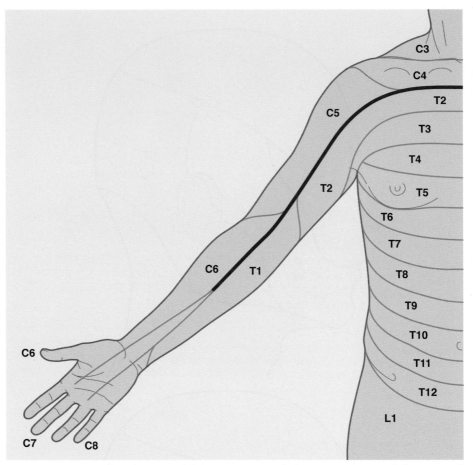

Fig. 93 Approximate distribution of dermatomes on the anterior aspect of the upper limb.

Figs 93–97 show the approximate cutaneous areas supplied by each spinal root. There is considerable variation and overlap between dermatomes, so that an isolated root lesion results in a much smaller area of sensory impairment than is indicated in these diagrams. The heavy axial lines are usually more consistent, showing the boundary between nonconsecutive dermatomes.

This variation also applies to the innervation of the fingers, but the thumb is usually supplied by C6 and the little finger by C8.

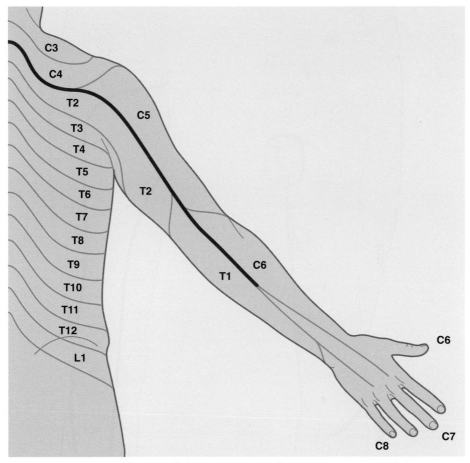

Fig. 94 Approximate distribution of dermatomes on the posterior aspect of the upper limb.

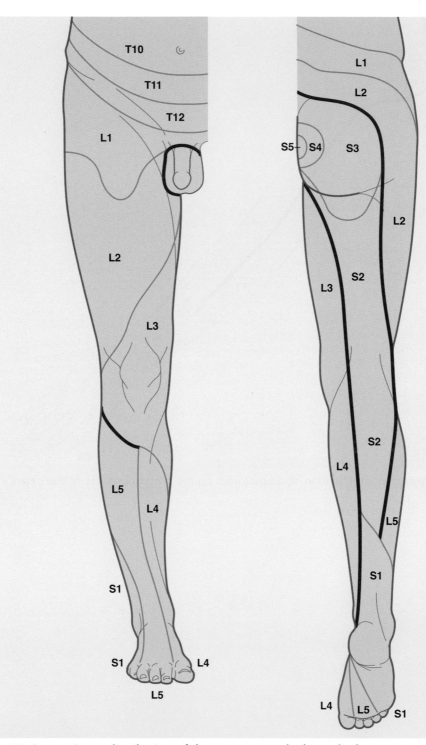

Fig. 95 Approximate distribution of dermatomes on the lower limb.

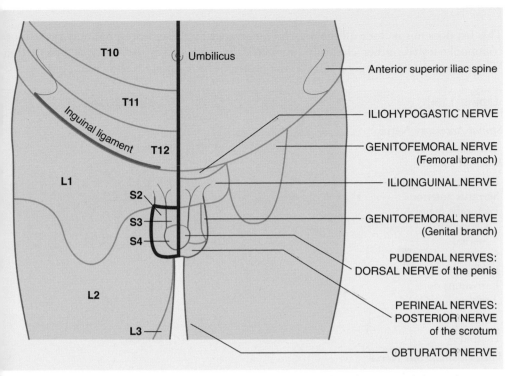

Fig. 96 Approximate distribution of dermatomes and peripheral nerves of the male inguinal region.

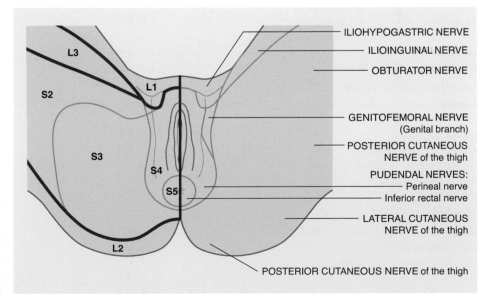

Fig. 97 Approximate distribution of dermatomes and peripheral nerves of the female perineum.

NERVE AND MAIN ROOT SUPPLY OF MUSCLES

This list does not include all the muscles innervated by these nerves, but only those more commonly tested, either clinically or electrically, and shows the order of innervation. Where several roots supply a muscle, the principal root supply is shown in bold.

Upper Limb	Spinal Roots
Spinal Accessory Nerve	
Trapezius	C3, **C4**
Brachial Plexus	
Rhomboids	C4, C5
Serratus anterior	C5, **C6**, C7
Pectoralis major	
Clavicular	C5, C6
Sternal	C6, **C7**, C8, T1
Supraspinatus	C5, C6
Infraspinatus	C5, C6
Latissimus dorsi	C6, **C7**
Teres major	C5, C6, C7
Axillary Nerve	
Deltoid	**C5**, C6
Musculocutaneous Nerve	
Biceps	**C5**, C6
Brachialis	C5, **C6**, C7
Radial Nerve	
Triceps {Long head, Lateral head, Medial head}	C6, **C7**, C8
Brachioradialis	C5, **C6**
Extensor carpi radialis longus	C5, **C6**
Posterior Interosseous Nerve	
Supinator	C6, C7
Extensor carpi ulnaris	C7, C8
Extensor digitorum	C7, C8
Abductor pollicis longus	C7, C8
Extensor pollicis longus	C7, C8
Extensor pollicis brevis	C7, C8
Extensor indicis	C7, C8
Median Nerve	
Pronator teres	C6, **C7**
Flexor carpi radialis	C6, **C7**
Flexor digitorum superficialis	C7, **C8**, T1
Abductor pollicis brevis	C8, **T1**
Flexor pollicis brevis*	C8, **T1**
Opponens pollicis	C8, **T1**
Lumbricals I and II	C8, **T1**

Anterior Interosseous Nerve

Pronator quadratus	C7, **C8**
Flexor digitorum profundus I and II	C7, **C8**
Flexor pollicis longus	C7, **C8**

Ulnar Nerve

Flexor carpi ulnaris	C7, **C8**
Flexor digitorum profundus III and IV	C7, **C8**
Hypothenar muscles	**C8**, T1
Adductor pollicis	**C8**, T1
Flexor pollicis brevis*	**C8**, T1
Palmar interossei	**C8**, T1
Dorsal interossei	**C8**, T1
Lumbricals III and IV	**C8**, T1

Lower Limb   Spinal Roots

Femoral Nerve

Iliopsoas	L1, **L2, L3**
Rectus femoris ⎫	
Vastus lateralis ⎬ Quadriceps femoris	L2, **L3, L4**
Vastus intermedius	
Vastus medialis ⎭	

Obturator Nerve

Adductor longus ⎫	L2, **L3, L4**
Adductor magnus ⎭	

Superior Gluteal Nerve

Gluteus medius and minimus ⎫	**L4, L5**, S1
Tensor fasciae latae ⎭	

Inferior Gluteal Nerve

Gluteus maximus	**L5, S1**, S2

Sciatic and Tibial Nerves

Semitendinosus	L5, **S1, S2**
Biceps	L5, **S1, S2**
Semimembranosus	L5, **S1, S2**
Gastrocnemius and Soleus	S1, S2
Tibialis posterior	L4, L5
Flexor digitorum longus	L5, **S1, S2**
Abductor hallucis ⎫	
Abductor digiti minimi ⎬ Small muscles of foot	S1, S2
Interossei ⎭	

Sciatic and Fibular Nerves

Tibialis anterior	**L4, L5**
Extensor digitorum longus	**L5**
Extensor hallucis longus	**L5**
Extensor digitorum brevis	**L5, S1**
Fibularis longus	**L5, S1**
Fibularis brevis	**L5, S1**

Flexor pollicis brevis is often supplied wholly or partially by the ulnar nerve.

COMMONLY TESTED MOVEMENTS

Movement	UMN	Root	Reflex	Nerve	Muscle
Upper Limb					
Shoulder abduction	++	C5		Axillary	Deltoid
Elbow flexion		C5, C6	+	Musculocutaneous	Biceps
		C6	+	Radial	Brachioradialis
Elbow extension	+	C7	+	Radial	Triceps
Radial wrist extension	+	C6		Radial	Extensor carpi radialis longus
Finger extension	+	C7		Posterior interosseus	Extensor digitorum communis
Finger flexion		C8	+	Anterior interosseus	Flexor pollicis longus
					Flexor digitorum profundus (index finger)
				Ulnar	Flexor digitorum profundus (ring and little fingers)
				Median	All other flexors
Finger abduction	++	T1		Ulnar	First dorsal interosseus
				Median	Abductor pollicis brevis
Lower Limb					
Hip flexion	++	L1, L2			Iliopsoas
Hip adduction		L2, L3	+	Obturator	Adductors
Hip extension		L5, S1		Sciatic	Gluteus maximus
Knee flexion	+	S1		Sciatic	Hamstrings
Knee extension		L3, L4	+	Femoral	Quadriceps
Ankle dorsiflexion	++	L4		Deep fibular	Tibialis anterior
Ankle eversion		L5, S1		Superficial fibular	Fibulares
Ankle plantarflexion		S1, S2	+	Tibial	Gastrocnemius, soleus
Ankle inversion		L4, L5		Tibial	Tibialis posterior
Big toe extension		L5	Babinski	Deep fibular	Extensor hallucis longus

The table shows some commonly tested movements, the principal muscle involved with the main roots and nerve supply. The column headed UMN indicates those movements that are evidently weaker in upper motor neuron lesions.